D1009478

Hormone Balance Through Yoga

A POCKET GUIDE FOR WOMEN OVER 40

CLAUDIA TURSKE

Hunter House
PUBLISHERS

German edition © 2010 by nymphenburger in der F.A.
Herbig Verlagsbuchhandlung GmbH, München
Original title: *Hormonbalance durch Yoga* • www.herbig.net
U.S. edition and translation © 2011 by Hunter House Inc., Publishers

All rights reserved. No part of this publication may be reproduced or transmitted in any form or by any means, electronic or mechanical, including photocopying and recording, or introduced into any information storage and retrieval system without the written permission of the copyright owner and the publisher of this book. Brief quotations may be used in reviews prepared for inclusion in a magazine, newspaper, or for broadcast. For further information please contact:

Hunter House Inc., Publishers
PO Box 2914, Alameda CA 94501-0914

Library of Congress Cataloging-in-Publication Data
Turske, Claudia, 1953–
[Hormonbalance durch Yoga. English]
Hormone balance through yoga : a pocket guide for women over 40 /
Claudia Turske. — 1st ed.
p. cm.
Includes index.
ISBN 978-0-89793-572-2 (pbk.)
1. Menopause—Popular works.   2. Middle-aged women—Health and hygiene.
3. Hormones—Popular works.   4. Hatha yoga—Therapeutic use.   I. Title.
RG186.T8713 2011
618.1'75—dc22   2011012081

Project Credits
Interior Photos: Jenny Sieboldt Fotografie, Berlin
Author Photo: Uwe Böhm
Illustrations: grudengrafik, Berlin

Cover Design: Brian Dittmar Design, Inc.	Acquisitions Assistant: Elizabeth Kracht
Book Production: John McKercher	Senior Marketing Associate: Reina Santana
Translator: Emily Banwell	Publicity & Marketing: Sean Harvey
Copy Editor: Amy Bauman	Rights Coordinator: Candace Groskreutz
Proofreader: John David Marion	Order Fulfillment: Washul Lakdhon
Managing Editor: Alexandra Mummery	Administrator: Theresa Nelson

Customer Service Manager: Christina Sverdrup
Computer Support: Peter Eichelberger
Publisher: Kiran S. Rana

Printed and bound by Bang Printing, Brainerd, Minnesota
Manufactured in the United States of America

9 8 7 6 5 4 3 2 1   First Edition   11 12 13 14 15

SACRAMENTO PUBLIC LIBRARY
828 "I" Street
Sacramento, CA 95814
9/11

Hormone Balance Through Yoga

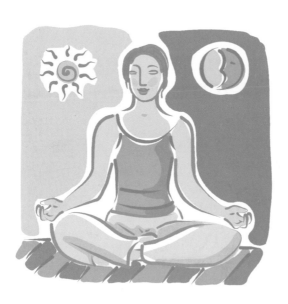

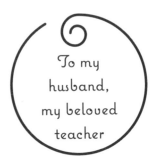

To my
husband,
my beloved
teacher

Ordering

Trade bookstores in the U.S. and Canada please contact:

Publishers Group West
1700 Fourth Street, Berkeley CA 94710
Phone: (800) 788-3123   Fax: (800) 351-5073

Hunter House books are available at bulk discounts for textbook course
adoptions; to qualifying community, health-care, and government
organizations; and for special promotions and fund-raising.
For details please contact:

Special Sales Department
Hunter House Inc., PO Box 2914, Alameda CA 94501-0914
Phone: (510) 865-5282   Fax: (510) 865-4295
E-mail: ordering@hunterhouse.com

Individuals can order our books from most bookstores,
by calling **(800) 266-5592**, or from our website at
www.hunterhouse.com

Contents

Important Note

The material in this book is intended to provide a review of information regarding hormone balance through the practice of yoga. The exercises presented in this book have been carefully tested by the author and have proven themselves in practice. Every effort has been made to provide accurate and dependable information, and the contents of this book have been compiled through professional research and in consultation with medical professionals. However, always consult your doctor or physical therapy practitioner before undertaking a new exercise regimen or doing any of the exercises or suggestions contained in this book. And in the event of any discomfort, please consult a doctor or other registered health practitioner.

The author, publisher, editors, and professionals quoted in the book cannot be held responsible for any error, omission, or dated material in the book. The author and publisher are not liable for any damage or injury or other adverse outcome of applying the information in this book in an exercise program carried out independently or under the care of a licensed trainer or practitioner. If you have questions concerning the application of the information described in this book, consult a qualified and trained professional.

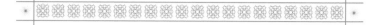

Preface

Dear women,

In this book I want to introduce you to some yoga exercises that helped me first reduce my menopause symptoms and then finally escape them altogether. Despite my long, intensive daily yoga practice, menopause changed my life so dramatically starting at age fifty-three that it was an effort just to get through my day-to-day tasks. Even teaching yoga classes became a burden. Only when I began to focus on specific hormone yoga exercises did I start to regain my original levels of energy and vitality.

Regain your energy and vitality.

Regaining Energy and Vitality

This guide is intended to help you practice at home. It grew out of my own need for guidance and has been refined over the years. I would like to thank everyone who supported me by providing me with feedback and commentary during these last few years of teaching and researching.

I owe a great deal to Dinah Rodrigues, who originally popularized this form of therapy; she inspired me to start learning more about this type of yoga practice, which is different from any other kind. In the process, I have made many changes and additional developments. I realized that using precise principles of biomechanical alignment (for instance, striving for an exact placement of the feet and pelvis, refining the way arms and legs are integrated into the shoulder and hip joints, examining the position of the head in relation to the torso, balancing the pelvis in relation to the thighs and knee joints) can make the complex movement sequences in yoga exercises much easier. Following these principles of alignment not only helps relieve existing pain in the back, knee joints, and shoulder joints, but it also helps prevent some of the injuries that commonly occur during yoga.

Hormone yoga reduces discomfort.

For many reasons, hormone yoga therapy is a sensible way of working with your own body. For one thing, it can significantly reduce menopause-related discomfort. It also counteracts hormonal imbalances and the resulting side effects.

However, the exercises also promote overall flexibility—both in a physical sense and a mental sense. Some of them are good for alleviating stress and preventing sleep disturbances, while others simply put you in a better mood and make you glad to be alive. Regular practice is a good idea in any case.

And with that I'd like to wish all of you sisters-in-arms and strong women much success—including great health and peace of mind—with your yoga practice.

CHAPTER 1

The Endocrine System

Hormones are active agents. They carry signals and messages throughout the body, regulating important biological functions, and they influence human responses and behaviors.

Hormones are created by the endocrine glands and distributed through the bloodstream. A key regulatory role is played by the hypothalamus and the pituitary gland in the lower section of the central brain (diencephalon).

The pea-sized pituitary gland produces ten main hormones. Four of these interact with the other endocrine glands, including the thyroid, which produces its own hormones. Also directly influenced by the pituitary gland are the adrenal glands, whose hormones affect stress responses, fluid levels, and kidney

Hormones influence responses and behaviors.

THE ENDOCRINE SYSTEM

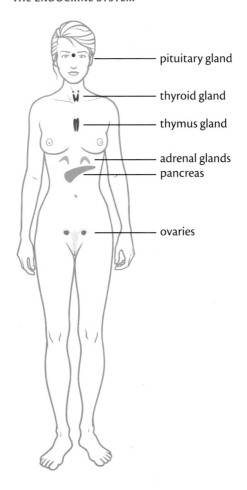

pituitary gland

thyroid gland

thymus gland

adrenal glands
pancreas

ovaries

function. The sex hormones, such as estrogen and progesterone in women, are produced by the sexual organs; they control the sex drive and initiate the responses associated with reproduction. If hormone production is irregular, the pituitary control center sends out messengers to restore balance.

Starting at age thirty-five, the production of estrogen very gradually begins to slow down. Between the ages of forty and fifty, this becomes very noticeable, and the end of menstruation indicates the start of menopause. Because of the sharp hormone fluctuations, many women experience a significant change for the worse in terms of mood and general well-being. As a result, this midlife phase is often not experienced as an enrichment but, rather, as a great burden. The severity of discomfort varies from one woman to the next, and it depends both on her physical and emotional characteristics and her circumstances.

Some Common Symptoms of Menopause

- nervousness and anxiety
- tiredness and listlessness
- hot flashes
- sweating
- dizziness
- depression
- joint pain and headaches
- hair loss
- brittle nails
- osteoporosis
- vaginal dryness
- decreased libido

(cont'd.)

Some Common Symptoms of Menopause (cont'd.)

- chronic musculoskeletal pain
- sleep disturbances and sleeplessness
- forgetfulness and lack of concentration

Overall, the process of hormonal change during menopause, the time when the female body is in transformation, can last about ten years.

The Phases of Menopause

Pre-menopause	the time when periods become irregular
Menopause	the time starting with the last menstrual period
Postmenopause	the time after menopause, which begins twelve months after the last menstrual period

During menopause, yoga can help prevent discomfort and provide women with ways to help lessen the symptoms. The active yoga exercises presented in this book work directly on the ovaries, the adrenal glands, and the thyroid through internal massage. In addition, intense mental concentration allows you to carry out the exercises on an energetic level, exerting a positive influence on the control center in your brain. A great deal of evidence now indicates that breathing and yoga exercises can have a positive effect (among others, see Jon Kabat-Zinn's studies on mindfulness-based stress reduction, or MBSR). It should be noted, though, that constant stress will neutralize any exercises you might be doing.

Stress causes excess adrenaline and norepinephrine to be released, which can have lasting health effects. Stress also is considered one of the causes of hormone imbalance, which is especially noticeable during menopause.[1] If even minor things stress you out, you lose the ability to regulate your moods.

So it is a good idea to pay attention to the extra breathing and concentration exercises for spiritual calmness. Schedule plenty of time for those exercises as well.

Stress affects hormone balance.

The results are surprisingly beneficial: We feel more energized and ready to tackle everyday tasks with confidence and optimism. In addition, a regular asana practice (in yoga, *asana* means "position" or "exercise") can restore physical flexibility and agility, making you look and feel young and radiant.

---

[1] Holsboer, Florian. 1993. "Stress und Hormone." *Spektrum der Wissenschaft*, 97. http://www.spektrumverlag.de/artikel/820829.

CHAPTER 2

The Basis: Breath and Energy

In yoga, breathing is a central component of the exercises and the practice. However, yogic breathing is also complex, and in its concentrated form, it can take great skill to master.

Breathing Techniques

Pranayama describes the breathing exercises used in yoga, and it teaches us how to use our inhalations, exhalations, and the pauses between them in a meaningful and energizing way.

Conscious breathing is energizing.

Prana means "breath, life, energy, and strength." *Ayama* means "stretching or expanding." Thus, *Pranayama* means extending the breath or one's life. B. K. S. Iyengar, probably the best-known teacher of Pranayama, writes: "Pranayama is an art and has techniques to make the respiratory organs to move and expand intentionally, rhythmically, and intensively. (...) [T]aking in plenty of oxygen while following these techniques in a disciplined way will create subtle chemical changes in the body."[1]

If you consciously use and regulate your breathing, it can also regulate your brain function and central nervous system. This in turn increases hormone production and the release of hormones, which can ease the symptoms of menopause.

Preliminary Exercise: Abdominal Breathing

In yoga, breathing primarily takes place through the nose. This makes the breath more controlled and regular. Deepening the breath causes what is known as abdominal breathing. As you inhale, the lowering of the diaphragm presses your abdominal wall outward; as you exhale, the diaphragm lifts and your abdominal wall moves backward. These movements very gently massage your internal organs, which has a stimulating and energizing effect.

The inner organs are gently massaged.

As an introduction, and as an easy way to practice abdominal breathing, lie on your back on the yoga mat and support your upper back with a folded blanket. Without pressure, breathe in and out through your nose; lay your hands flat on

[1] Iyengar, B. K. S. 2008. *Light on Pranayama*. New York: HarperCollins.

your abdomen, palms down. Taking your time, close your eyes and gently turn your attention inward; you will notice that your breath grows deeper and more regular. If you listen carefully, you will discover a very faint sound that is beautiful and calming. If this exercise comes easily, sit on a blanket or a firm pillow with your legs crossed. Close your eyes, place one hand on your abdomen below the navel, and breathe deeply so that your hand starts to move as your abdominal wall expands and contracts. Once again, listen carefully and discover the regular sound of your breathing.

If it is difficult to do this exercise while seated, you can use a strap to assist you. Place the strap loosely around your lower ribs. Breathing calmly through your nose and with your eyes closed, you will notice how the abdominal breathing works. As you breathe in, your rib cage steadily expands, the strap grows tighter, and your abdominal wall expands. As you breathe out, the abdominal wall and rib cage return to their original position.

Ujjayi Pranayama (Ocean Breath)

Ujjayi means "victoriously uprising" or "victory from expansion."[2] It refers to the energy that is created by deep, regulated breathing, which then rises and expands.

[2] Keller, Doug. 2003. *Refining the Breath.* 2nd ed, 39. South Riding, VA: Do Yoga Productions.

Ujjayi has two main characteristics: The first is its deep regularity, and the second is the quiet sound that is created by narrowing the glottis. In our exercises, the main function of Ujjayi Pranayama, in addition to concentration and awareness, is to massage the thyroid gland.

You can practice audible breathing by opening your mouth and breathing out with a "haaaaaaa" sound (as if you were breathing on a mirror or on your glasses to clean them). In doing so, you will discover that your glottis contracts. If you do the same thing with your lips closed, it creates a clearly audible, slight hissing noise. The air flowing in and out is channeled and regulated, and the vibration gently massages your larynx and thyroid.

Ujjayi breathing creates concentration and awareness.

Agni Bhastrika Pranayama (Bellows Breath; Bhastrika Breathing)

Agni Bhastrika Pranayama, or Bhastrika breathing, is also described as the "bellows breath" (*agni* means "fire," and the *bhastrika*, or "bellows," is used to fan the flames). Take fast, short, deep breaths into your belly until your abdominal wall lifts; breathing out quickly, actively draw in your belly so that your navel is pulled toward your spine. Do not move your rib cage as you breathe. This breath takes place exclusively in the belly. Both the in and the out breath should be strong and powerful, creating a sound like a bellows.

Bhastrika creates a large amount of energy (*prana*) and activates the entire body. In our exercises, the main purpose of Bhastrika, other than providing energy, is to massage the ovaries through the strong movement of the abdominal wall.

The entire body is activated.

The best way to practice this technique is to do so while lying on your belly. In this position, even if you breathe more quickly, it is easy to feel the abdominal wall expanding as you breathe in and moving back toward the spine as you breathe out.

Technique for Directing Energy Within the Body

The six steps for directing energy make up the most important technique that we use in hormone-balancing yoga. It is a good idea to learn this sequence by heart, because it is used in almost every exercise:

1. Breathe in and then pause. Close your eyes.

2. With your eyes closed, focus on the tip of your nose. (In yoga, this is called single-pointed focus, or *eka grata*. It makes the spirit highly concentrated, and if you focus on a single point, you will not be distracted.)

3. Roll the tip of your tongue inward and place it against the roof of your mouth to hold the upward-moving energy inside your head.

4. Then practice Mula Bandha (see below) to hold the downward energy inside your pelvis.

5. Life energy (prana) will then rise up along your spine to the tip of your nose.

6. Direct your concentration toward the endocrine gland (the thyroid or ovaries, for instance) that you want to activate in the exercise and calmly breathe out.

The technique sounds very complex here, but it actually takes only a few seconds to perform. Breathing in, concentrating on the tip of your nose, and rolling your tongue all happen at the same time; practicing Mula Bandha and concentrating on the desired endocrine gland takes one to two seconds; and breathing out (while tracing the sensation) concludes the process of directing your energy.

Practicing Mula Bandha (Root Chakra Lock; Pelvic Floor Lock or Sustained Contraction)

All together, there are three bandhas. These are targeted soft muscle contractions that help steer the flow of energy. In Mula Bandha, gently contract the muscles of the perineum while simultaneously moving your tailbone down and forward in a shoveling motion by tipping your pelvis. This creates a kind of sluice that gathers the energy in the pelvic floor and channels it.

The energy in the pelvic floor is channeled.

It is a good idea to practice Mula Bandha in front of a mirror a few times. Stand sideways in front of the mirror. Move your thighs backward slightly (so you look as though you have a sort of ducktail) and place one hand on your tailbone. Place your other hand on your belly, just over the pubic bone. Now tip your pelvis without moving your thighs—the hand on your back will move downward, and the front hand will move upward.

Note: *Mula Bandha should not be practiced too vigorously or the muscles in the anus will contract, which can cause hemorrhoids.*

CHAPTER 3

Warm-Up Exercises

It is important to prepare your body, to warm it up, before you begin the daily exercises. This helps prevent injuries. The following nine warm-up exercises will loosen areas of tension and start stimulating hormone production.

If you have time, it is ideal to do all of the warm-up exercises before starting the daily exercise program. If you practice daily, you will sooner or later be flexible enough that you will be able to choose just a few warm-up exercises for the body parts that need it most.

Warming up the body is essential.

Preparation

Wear loose exercise pants and a cotton T-shirt.

Always practice barefoot on a yoga mat so that you don't slip.

You will need a few additional props for your practice:

* a block (or two blocks, if you can't touch the ground with your hands in a forward bend)
* a strap
* a blanket
* a meditation cushion or a small, firm pillow

Loosening the Shoulders

Starting position: Place your feet hip-distance apart. Stand upright.

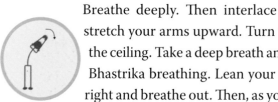

Breathe deeply, interlace your fingers, and stretch your arms upward. Turn your palms to face the ceiling. Take a deep breath and begin to practice Bhastrika breathing (see page 9) as follows: As you breathe in, lift your arms, and as you breathe out, lower them. Repeat this exercise seven to fifteen times.

Side Bends

Starting position: Place your feet hip-distance apart. Stand upright.

Breathe deeply. Then interlace your fingers and stretch your arms upward. Turn your palms to face the ceiling. Take a deep breath and begin to practice Bhastrika breathing. Lean your upper body to the right and breathe out. Then, as you breathe in, bring your body back to the center. Make sure your torso does not move forward or backward as you bend from side to side. Repeat the exercise seven to fifteen times on the right side. Then do the same exercise on the left side.

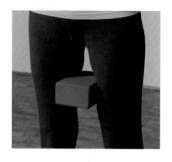

TIP: Holding a block between your thighs will help you keep your pelvis in the starting position.

Chest Opener

Starting position: Place your feet hip-distance apart. Stand upright.

Breathe deeply. Then reach your arms behind you and interlace your fingers (keeping the palms apart). Draw your shoulders upward and backward, shoulder blades together, and make sure not to overextend your elbows.

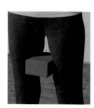
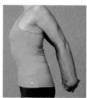
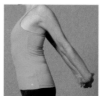

Practice Bhastrika breathing: Breathe in as you draw your hands backward and breathe out as you bring them back toward your sacrum. Repeat the exercise seven to fifteen times.

TIP: Your head will involuntarily move forward, so keep the back of your head tall and draw it backward. In order to keep your upright stance and stability in your feet and legs, you can place a block between your thighs.

Swinging the Hips—Loosening the Pelvis

Starting position: Place your feet in a parallel position, 8 to 12 inches apart, with your knees slightly bent.

Lift your arms above your shoulders and clasp your fingers at the nape of your neck. Breathe deeply and then practice Bhastrika breathing while swinging your hips from side to side. Start in the center position, breathing in, and then breathe out as you swing to the right. Breathe in as you return to the center, then breathe out as you swing to the right again. Repeat the exercise seven to fifteen times. Repeat the exercise to the other side: Breathe in from the center and breathe out as you move to the left. Breathe in as you return to the center, breathe out as you move to the left.

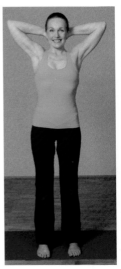 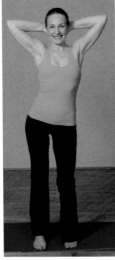 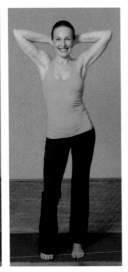

TIP: Keep your knees loose.

Mobilizing the Spine

Starting position: Place your feet hip-distance apart. Stand upright.

Breathe deeply and bend your knees while pushing your pelvis and your buttocks backward. Place your palms on your knees to support yourself. Make sure your fingers are pointing downward (don't turn your hands inward). Take a breath and hold it. Still holding your breath, move your rib cage forward and

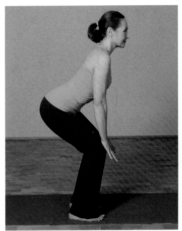 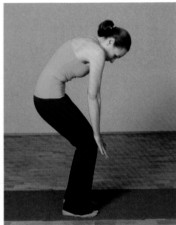

backward in a wavelike motion, as many times as you can do so without feeling pressure from holding your breath. Keep your arms extended. This exercise activates the adrenal glands, the thymus gland, and the pancreas.

Repeat the exercise a total of three times, inhaling and exhaling completely between each repetition.

TIP: To hold your breath longer, fill your lungs only three-quarters of the way full when you breathe in.

Standing Leg Stretch and Balancing Exercise
Starting position: Place your feet hip-distance apart. Stand upright.

Breathe deeply. Then bend your right knee and draw it upward toward your chest; clasp your shin with both hands and hold your torso upright.

Take three Ujjayi breaths (see page 8) to help stretch out your back muscles. Once your stance feels stable, hold onto the outer edge of your foot with your right hand, slowly stretch your right leg out in front of you, and then move it to the side. Take three more Ujjayi breaths. Finally, repeat the whole sequence on the left side.

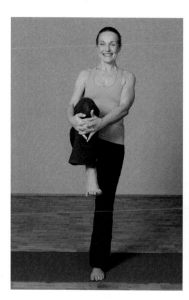
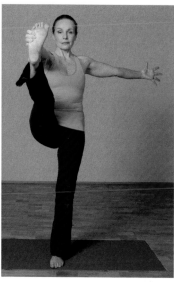

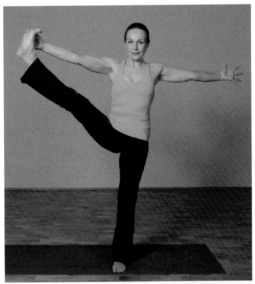

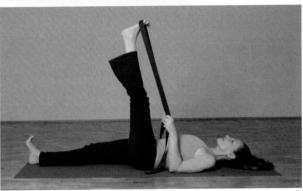

TIP: If you have trouble keeping your balance, you can hold onto the wall with your other hand for support. If you have a slipped disk or other back problems, do this exercise lying down, using a strap to hold your foot, until your muscles are elongated and fully stretched out. If you practice frequently, becoming more flexible will take just a few weeks!

Stretching the Hamstrings and Torso

Starting position: Place your feet hip-distance apart. Stand upright.

Breathe deeply. Bend forward and place your fingertips on the mat (or other surface) under your shoulders. You can also use two blocks if your fingertips

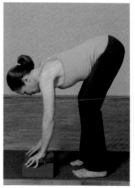 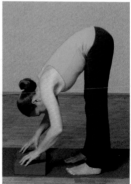 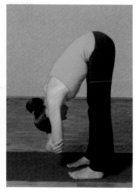

don't yet reach the ground. Breathe deeply. Place your right hand on your left elbow and your left hand on your right elbow. Let your head hang down loosely.

Practice seven to fifteen Bhastrika breaths and repeat the entire sequence three times.

Increasing Hip Flexibility, Stretching the Achilles Tendon
Starting position: Place your feet hip-distance apart. Stand upright.

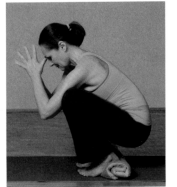

Take a deep breath. As you breathe out, squat down and bring your palms together in front of your chest. Place your upper arms on the insides of your knees. You can use this resistance to straighten your back while gently drawing your shoulder blades together.

While in this deep squat, practice seven to fifteen Bhastrika breaths.

TIP: If your heels don't reach the floor in this position, place a rolled-up blanket underneath them for support.

Increasing Upper-Spine Flexibility

Starting position: Sit down with your legs crossed and your spine straight. Use your hands to pull your buttocks backward and apart so that you are sitting firmly on your sitting bones.

Interlace your fingers in front of your chest and lift your elbows to shoulder height. Keep your eyes open and focus on your hands; breathe deeply. Then practice Bhastrika breathing as follows: As you breathe out, quickly swing your upper body to the right, moving your head in the same direction. As you breathe in, turn your body back to the center (with enough energy to flip your hair).

Repeat the exercise seven to fifteen times on the right side and then switch to the left side.

TIP: If you can't hold your back straight, sit on a folded blanket. If you have a slipped disk, sit on the front edge of a chair.

CHAPTER 4

Exercises for Hormonal Balance

This daily sequence of exercises should be practiced until the exercises have become second nature. If you don't have any experience with daily practice, allow plenty of time at first (ninety minutes). Your personal attitude is equally important. Hormone yoga works when you practice it regularly. Put yourself in the role of a curious child and observe the changes that result. This will make your practice playful and fun. Once you have done the exercises often enough, 35 minutes should be enough time to go through the daily sequence.

A few suggestions for your own practice:

Practice playfully and joyfully; be curious like a little child.

* If you are suffering from the full range of menopausal symptoms, it is a good idea to practice daily until you experience relief. You can see for yourself how much the exercises are helping, and if you fill in the calendar (see page 54) you may also discover that three or four sessions a week are enough to maintain your sense of well-being.

* If you are suffering only from an underactive thyroid, for instance, you can reduce the exercises that treat the ovaries and concentrate more on the thyroid exercises.

* If you are feeling very stressed, concentrate on the breathing exercises; these will help you better manage the challenges in your life.

After a while, the exercise program will evolve into your own personal well-being program, and you can focus on the exercises that feel best for you.

Adho Muka Svanasana (Downward-Facing Dog)

Starting position: Start on all fours with your hands shoulder-distance apart and your feet and knees hip-distance apart. Curl your toes under. Gently breathe in and out: Your practice begins.

Move your knees backward about 6 inches. Making sure your hands and feet are well grounded, draw your pelvis upward and gently pull your shoulder blades together. Leave your knees slightly bent. Spread out your fingers and press into your fingertips to powerfully stretch your arms. (Be careful not to hyperextend your elbows.) Rotate your upper thighs inward, backward, and apart, keeping your back long, and push your buttocks upward. Then, slowly stretch your legs and pull your tailbone downward until your heels are on or near the floor. Your gaze

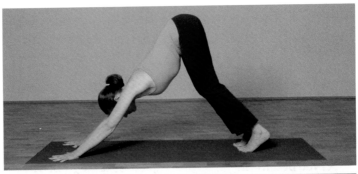

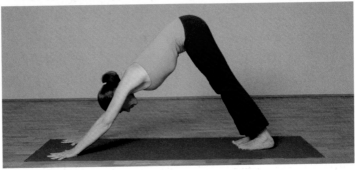

should be directed downward and your neck should stay long. Take three deep and long Ujjayi breaths in this position.

TIP: To determine how much distance should be between your hands and your feet, start on your hands and knees and then get into position to do a push-up (also known as plank position). This distance should not change during the exercise.

This position opens up both your shoulders and pelvis, stretches the sides of your body, and creates a deep sense of awareness for what will come next.

Lunge

Starting position: Adho Muka Svanasana (Downward-Facing Dog) as described on pages 25–27.

As you breathe in, place your right foot at the front of the mat between your hands. Your right knee should be positioned directly over the ankle joint. Stretch out your left leg, with your left toes pressing into the ground. Your shoulder blades should lie flat against your back, and your back should stay long and straight.

Take seven to fifteen Bhastrika breaths in this position and then direct your energy to your right ovary (see "Technique for Directing Energy Within the Body" on page 10).

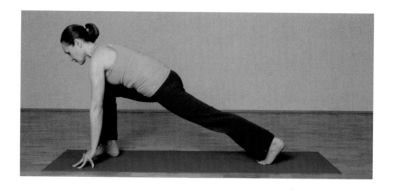

Finally, move your right foot backward to match the left foot and take three deep Ujjayi breaths in Adho Muka Svanasana (Downward-Facing Dog).

Repeat the exercise with your left foot.

This exercise massages the ovaries (right and left), which stimulates hormone production in the ovaries.

Eka Pada Rajakapotasana (Pigeon Pose)

Starting position: As shown below.

Your right heel should be near the left side of your groin with the knee pointing forward. Your left leg stretches straight backward. Curl the toes on your left foot under and make sure your pelvis is straight. Your upper body should lean out over your front leg, and your arms should be extended.

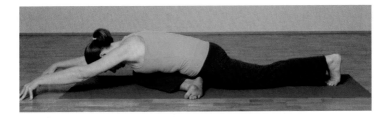

Take seven to fifteen Bhastrika breaths and then direct your energy to the right ovary (see "Technique for Directing Energy Within the Body" on page 10).

Repeat the exercise two more times on the right side; then switch positions so that your upper body is leaning over your left leg and repeat the exercise three more times.

This exercise massages the ovaries (right and left), which stimulates their production of hormones.

Supta Virasana (Reclining Hero Pose) Variation

Starting position: Lie flat on your back. Bend your knees and place the soles of your feet on the floor. Now lift your pelvis and place a folded blanket under your sacrum. Cross your lower legs and sink your knees down toward the floor (in an easy lotus position). Reach your arms out over your head and interlace your fingers with your palms facing outward. Your belly should remain taut and your pelvis slightly elevated. In this position, take seven to fifteen Bhastrika breaths and then

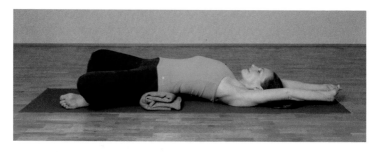

direct your energy to both ovaries at the same time. Repeat the sequence three more times.

Next create a vacuum in your lower body:

Keeping your hands clasped, bend your arms slightly and take a deep breath. As you breathe out, empty your lungs completely and extend your arms again. Once you have finished breathing out, draw your abdominal wall inward and upward. Hold this position as long as you can while holding your breath without pressure. Then let the air flow back into your lungs and release the vacuum.

Repeat the exercise two more times.

This exercise massages the ovaries (right and left), which stimulates their production of hormones.

Exercises for a Radiant Appearance:
"Beauty Waves" (from Dinah Rodrigues)
These exercises will make you glow and give you fresh energy.

The First Beauty Wave

Starting position: Lie flat on your back.

Bend both knees and draw your thighs in toward your belly; clasp your thighs with your arms.

Next take seven Bhastrika breaths before directing your energy to your face and hair (see "Technique for Directing Energy Within the Body" on page 10).

The Second Beauty Wave

Starting position: Lie on your back with your hands and wrists under your hips, palms facing down. Your thumbs should be touching.

Putting pressure on your wrists is extremely efficient because these pressure points help activate the ovaries.

Keep your wrists underneath your hips with your palms facing down. Reach your legs straight up to the ceiling and alternately kick your right and left heels against your buttocks while doing Bhastrika breathing (breathing out as you kick with your right foot and breathing in as you kick with

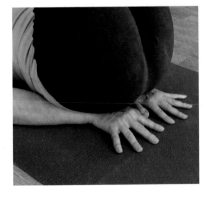

your left foot). After seven to fifteen kicks, you can direct your energy to your face and hair.

TIP: Keep your thighs vertical and your feet in a position that allows the heels to touch each side of the buttocks.

The Third Beauty Wave

Repeat the sequence, this time Bhastrika breathing out as you kick with your left foot and breathing in as you kick with your right foot. Place your feet back on the floor before freeing your wrists. Place your feet at the edges of the mat and let your knees fall together.

Feel the tickling sensation in your wrists and relax with a smile.

Setu Bandha Sarvangasana (Bridge Pose)

Starting position: Lie on your back with your knees bent. Place your feet hip-distance apart and parallel to one another, with your middle fingers touching your heels.

Draw your shoulder blades together against your back and relax your shoulders. Press the back of your head firmly into the mat with your neck lifted upward, off the floor. Start taking calm Ujjayi breaths to massage the thyroid.

As you breathe in using the Ujjayi technique, smoothly

lift your pelvis and your rib cage in a flowing motion. Then lower your rib cage and your pelvis back to the floor in a flowing motion, as you breathe out with an Ujjayi exhale.

Repeat this exercise seven times. Finish in the elevated position and support your pelvis with your hands or with a block.

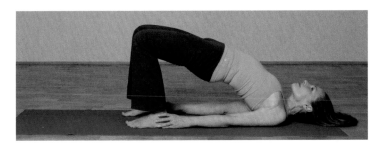

Stay in this position and take seven to fifteen Bhastrika breaths. Then lower your rib cage and pelvis back to the floor and direct your energy to your thyroid gland.

This exercise activates the thyroid gland and stimulates production of thyroid hormone.

Supta Tadasana (Reclined Mountain Pose)

Starting position: Lie on your back with your legs extended, hip-distance apart. Your toes should be pointing upward and spread apart, and your arms and hands should be extended alongside your upper body with the muscles engaged. While pressing the back of your head gently into the floor, pull your shoulders upward toward your ears and then gently draw your shoulder blades together against your back.

Now lift your head (not your shoulders) and look at your feet. Bend your chin toward your sternum without closing off your windpipe. Take three to five deep breaths using the Ujjayi technique, then direct your energy to your thyroid gland (see "Technique for Directing Energy Within the Body" on page 10).

This exercise helps you massage the right and left lobes of the thyroid, and it stimulates production of thyroid hormone.

Matsyasana (Fish Pose)

Starting position: Lie on your back with your legs extended hip-distance apart. Your toes should be pointing upward and spread apart. Put the palms of your hands under your buttocks and link your thumbs together. Press the back of your head gently into the floor to pull your shoulders upward toward your ears and then draw your shoulder blades together against your back.

Next firmly press your elbows and forearms into the floor and lift your upper body, supporting yourself on your forearms.

Lift your sternum toward the ceiling and slowly let your head sink back toward the floor.

Note: *Be careful not to put any pressure on your neck as you do this!*

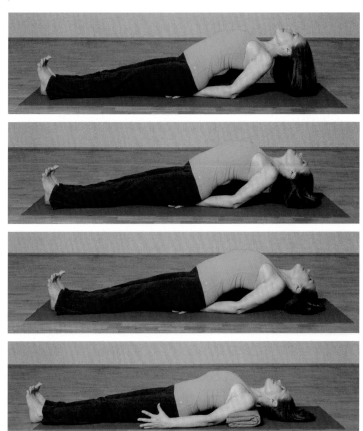

Take three Ujjayi breaths and then direct your energy to the thyroid (see "Technique for Directing Energy Within the Body" on page 10). This exercise also stimulates production of thyroid hormone.

TIP: If you have neck problems, it is a good idea to place a firm pillow (or a folded blanket) under your mid-back (approximately where your bra sits) instead of supporting yourself with your forearms. This allows your head to be supported by the floor. If the pillow is in the right place, you will feel a strong stretch in the neck region as you breathe out using the Ujjayi technique.

Janu Sirsasana (Head-to-Knee Pose)

Starting position: Sit upright on the floor with your legs spread wide apart. Your toes should be pointing toward the ceiling and spread apart. With your right hand, grasp the inside of your right thigh at the knee and bend your knee. With your left hand, hold the bottom of your right heel and place your foot in front of the pubic bone, with the top of your foot touching the floor. Your heel should be facing up. The angle between the two thighs should be at least 90 degrees.

Reach your arms up overhead and twist your upper body

toward your left leg. As you breathe in, extend your upper body and arms. As you breathe out, bend forward and hold onto your left foot.

Take seven Bhastrika breaths, pushing your foot forward as you breathe out and pulling it backward as you breathe in, with a motion similar to stepping on the gas pedal of a car. Next breathe in, keep your foot flexed, and direct your

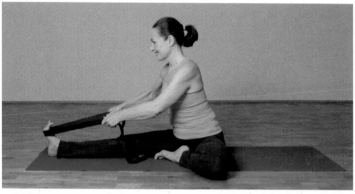

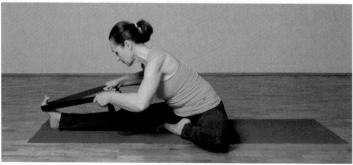

energy to your left ovary (see "Technique for Directing Energy Within the Body" on page 10).

Repeat the exercise on the other side of your body.

This exercise helps massage the ovaries (right and left), which stimulates their production of hormones.

TIP: If you cannot reach your foot, loop a strap around the ball of your foot (not the arch of the foot) to enable yourself to perform the exercise.

Ardha Matsyendrasana (Half Spinal Twist)

Starting position: Sit upright on the floor (sit on a folded blanket if your lower back does not curve inward as much as it should and you experience a dull ache in the lumbar region). Your legs should be extended; your toes should be pointing toward the ceiling and spread out.

Bend your left knee and place your left foot next to your right knee. Hold onto the bent knee with both hands and pull your back upward until you are sitting up tall and straight. Take seven Bhastrika breaths and then direct your energy to your left ovary (see "Technique for Directing Energy Within the Body" on page 10).

Next place your left foot on the outside of the extended right leg. Twist your rib cage to the left, holding onto the bent

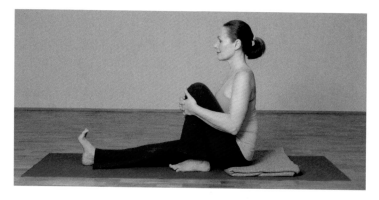

leg with your right arm. Draw your left shoulder up toward your ear and then pull your shoulder blades together on your back. Place the fingertips of your left hand on the floor behind your buttocks. As you breathe in, lengthen your upper body; as you breathe out, twist your spine and rib cage (not just your head). Take seven Bhastrika breaths and then direct

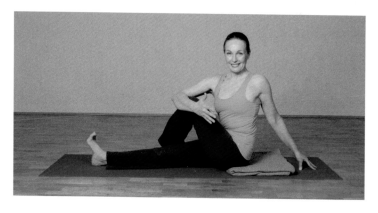

your energy to your right ovary (see "Technique for Directing Energy Within the Body" on page 10).

Twist your upper body even farther to the left, holding onto your extended right leg with your right hand. Your right elbow should be on the outside of your left knee (bend your left knee slightly less). Take seven Bhastrika breaths and then direct your energy to your left ovary.

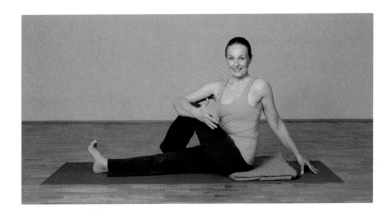

Repeat all three steps of this exercise on the left side.

This exercise helps massage the ovaries (right and left) and stimulates their production of hormones.

TIP: To protect your elbow joints, avoid hyperextending your arms.

Sarvangasana (Shoulder Stand)

NOTE: *The ideal duration for these three dynamic inversions is four to five minutes total. Repeat the sequence until the appropriate amount of time has passed. Slowly increase the time and don't give up if the exercises are hard at first. They will grow easier over time.*

To support your neck, place a blanket on the mat, folded into a square so that you can fold the top third of the mat back over the blanket (see photo).

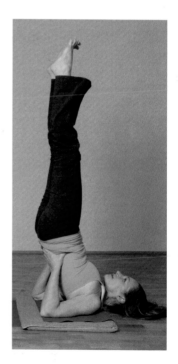

Starting position: Lie flat on your back. Your shoulders should be on the folded part of the mat, and your head should be on the floor. Bend your knees.

Bend your elbows and press them firmly into the floor. Draw your shoulder blades together against your back. Press the back of your head into the floor and pull your chin away from your sternum. Lift your legs and pelvis and support your hips with your hands, holding your thumbs at waist level in front of the hip bones. Stretch your legs as high up as possible, spreading your toes. Make sure that the nape of your neck stays off the ground. Take approximately fifteen Bhastrika breaths and direct your energy to the thyroid and pituitary glands. The next two exercises will also be carried out in this position; finish by directing your energy to the thyroid and pituitary glands.

TIP: If your wrists become too tired, you can lower your hips and relax your wrists by moving your hands in small circles. Then go back into the inversion and continue until you have spent four to five minutes total in the pose. If you have never done a shoulder stand before and you have trouble elevating your pelvis over your chest, you can place a thick cushion under your pelvis and lower back, creating a position that provides the inversion without the same amount of strain.

These exercises help drain the blood from the legs and improve the overall circulation of blood. They also activate the thyroid and pituitary glands, and regulate hormone balance.

Sarvangasana (Shoulder Stand) Variation 1
Starting position: Begin in Sarvangasana (described on the previous page). Extend your legs outward into a V-shape, without letting them tip forward.

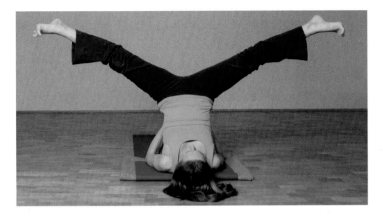

Try to relax your pelvic floor completely by taking calm, deep breaths.

Practice fifteen Bhastrika breaths in this position and pay attention to the movement of the perineum. Finally direct your energy to the thyroid and pituitary glands (see "Technique for Directing Energy Within the Body" on page 10).

This exercise will help you relax the pelvic floor and groin, thereby lessening constriction in the pelvic area.

Sarvangasana (Shoulder Stand) Variation 2

Starting position: Begin in Sarvangasana (described on page 41), in which the legs are extended together toward the ceiling.

Now take turns moving each extended leg toward your head and then backward, as if you were walking.

Practice Bhastrika breathing as follows: Breathe in as you move the right leg downward and breathe out as you move the left leg downward.

Direct your energy to the thyroid and pituitary glands (see "Technique for Directing Energy Within the Body" on page 10).

Repeat the exercise. This time breath out at the same time as the right leg moves downward and breath in as the left leg moves downward.

When coming out of the pose, loosely reach your legs backward and release your hands. Stretch your arms out on the mat and press down strongly with the palms of your hands. This allows you to control your pelvis and to slowly roll it down to the floor. Halfway down, you can bend your knees, which makes it easy to come out of this complex pose.

Windshield Wiper

Starting position: Lie flat on your back with your legs bent and your feet planted mat-distance apart—the outer edges of your feet are at the edge of the mat. Angle your arms up into a sort of "cactus pose," keeping your neck long.

As you breathe out, pull your right knee diagonally toward your left foot. The left leg stays upright.

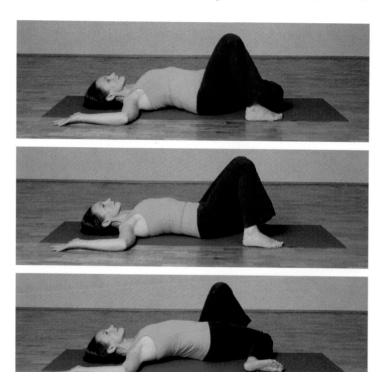

Lift your knee back upward as you breathe in. The next time you breathe out, pull your left knee diagonally toward your right ankle, keeping your right leg steady.

Repeat the exercise several times.

This exercise feels good after doing the shoulder stands, and it neutralizes the inversion poses.

Shavasana (Corpse Pose)

Starting position: Lie flat on your back. Spread your legs until your feet are mat-distance apart, let your feet and legs fall outward, and relax.

Extend your arms next to your upper body, draw your shoulder blades flat against your back, and turn your palms up. Keep your neck and throat long and keep your head placed heavy on the floor.

Direct your awareness to your inward center; carefully observe your breath as you exhale.

Mentally explore your body and your skin, starting with your head. Observe your bones, muscles, and joints and try to release tension. Through the use of your breath, release all of your weight into the floor. Borne by your breath, stay still for seven to ten minutes, but refrain from falling asleep.

Shavasana is the concluding pose in every yoga session. It relaxes the entire body and mind after a strenuous practice and helps provide a complete sense of regeneration.

TIP: If you wish, you can also use a blanket for Shavasana. The blanket should loosely cover your body without restricting it.

CHAPTER 5

Additional Exercises for Calming the Mind

One of the most effective ways to become calmer and fight stress is to practice Pranayama, or breathing exercises, on a daily basis. These exercises balance out our emotional responses.

It is very important to reduce stress, because it is one of the causes of hormone imbalance. Even if you don't have time to practice all of the hormone yoga exercises on a daily basis, it is still a good idea to do a few of the stress-reducing exercises at night before you go to sleep. These exercises can also be used to finish off the daily exercise regimen.

Breathing exercises have a calming effect.

Calming Pranayama

Starting position for all Pranayama exercises: When practicing Pranayama, always sit upright on a blanket or pillow, with your back straight, and have your legs crossed with your feet supporting your calves (see the illustration for Chandra Bhedana on page 50). If this is challenging for you, sit upright on the edge of a chair with your feet and legs placed hip-distance apart. Take the attitude of a neutral observer—as if you were sitting next to yourself and watching, without evaluation or judgment. This creates a pleasant distance: being present without being involved.

Breathe in while counting to three. Breathe out while counting to six. Do this exercise for a couple of minutes a day, increasing your breath count to four and eight or five and ten. Stop the exercise if breathing becomes difficult or your mind starts to wander.

Sama Vritti (Equal Breathing)

Starting position: Sit upright on a blanket with your buttocks on the ground and your legs crossed, your calves resting on your feet. Place your hands on your knees in a closed Jñana Mudra (breath regulation) position (see illustration).

Breathe in while counting to four. Then hold your breath

for another count of four. As you breathe out, count to four once again. And then count to four again before taking your next breath.

TIP: If you have circulatory problems or high blood pressure, leave out the step of holding your breath for a count of four (with your lungs full of air).

Nadi Shodhana (Alternate-Nostril Breathing)

Starting position: Take the same seated Pranayama starting position described in Sama Vritti (above). Place your left hand on your left knee.

Fold the index and middle finger of your right hand toward your palm. Your thumb and ring finger act as pincers, using very gentle pressure to alternately hold your right and left nostril closed. Keep your pinky finger positioned loosely next to your ring finger.

First take a few deep breaths into your belly as you get used to the grip on your nose. Then consciously breathe out. Start by closing your right nostril and breathing in through your left nostril. Then gently close your left nostril, release your right nostril, and breathe out.

Next reverse the move, breathing in through the right side and out through the left side.

Repeat the sequence as many times as you like. Finish by breathing out on the left side.

TIP: It is important to press lightly when closing your nostrils. Pressing too hard on the sides of the nose could impair sensitivity. The concentration involved in this exercise creates a calming effect, and it helps restore balance to the neurovegetative system.

Chandra Bhedana

Starting position: Take the same seated Pranayama starting position described in Sama Vritti (see page 48). Place your left hand on your left knee.

Chandra Bhedana is a Pranayama exercise in which you slowly inhale only through the left nostril and breathe out only through the right.

Form the Nadi Shodhana hand position shown on page 49, using your right hand. Gently hold your right nostril closed as you breathe in and your left nostril closed as you breathe out.

Do this exercise until you feel calm.

TIP: If you have trouble sleeping, you can also do this exercise in bed.

Soham

Starting position: While on a blanket, sit up on your knees with the backs of your thighs resting on the backs of your calves and the bottoms of your feet facing upward. Your legs can either be straight or crossed under you. If this is too painful, sit with your buttocks on the ground and your legs crossed, with your calves resting on your feet.

Bring both hands into Jñana Mudra position (see page 48) with your palms facing up. Straighten your right arm and lift it so the upper part of that arm is near your ear; your left arm should stay down by your knee. Lift your right arm, breathe in, and sing "SO" without moving. Then sing "HAM" while lowering the right arm and raising the left arm like a see-saw. Coordinate the movement so that it ends as you slowly finish singing "HAM."

Repeat this exercise as long as it feels good to do so.

To finish the exercise, lower your raised arm. Can you feel the energy moving through your arms? You may also feel a sense of balance and inner harmony.

Amritsa

Starting position: Take the same seated Pranayama starting position described in Sama Vritti (see page 48). Place your hands on your knees with your palms facing upward.

Now silently repeat the mantra "AM—RI—TSA" to yourself. As you do so, move your fingers along with your breathing as follows:

The thumb very quickly and gently touches first the index finger and then the middle finger and the ring finger as you breathe in. To yourself, repeat "AM—RI—TSA" in time with the fingers. As you breathe out, the thumb first touches the pinky finger, then the ring finger, and finally the middle finger. Again, repeat the mantra "AM—RI—TSA" as you breathe out. As you breathe in, start the sequence with the index finger again.

TIP: This exercise also helps with insomnia; it is like counting sheep.

Relaxing the Mind

Starting position: Lie on your back with your feet on the floor and your knees bent.

Bring your right foot close to your left buttock; place your left foot on your right knee. Let your propped-up left leg sink down to the right. As you grow more flexible, you will be able to move your knee closer and closer to the ground. Place your right hand on your left knee.

Now let your energy circulate in a counterclockwise direction. Start by focusing on your left hand, breathe in, and send the energy from your left hand to your throat. Breathe out while sending the energy to your right hand; then to your left knee, left foot, and right knee; back to your right foot; and finally to your left hand.

Repeat this exercise several times. Then slowly and carefully reverse your twisting direction before repeating the sequence on the other side of your body.

Once again, direct your energy counterclockwise, starting with your left hand, which should now be on your right knee.

CHAPTER 6

My Hormone Yoga Calendar

To note the efficiency of your hormone yoga practice, it is a good idea to mark down the days when you practice and to evaluate how you feel. This is the only way to tell how helpful your practice is. The following calendar will help you gain a clear and honest picture of your progress and recognize even small steps forward in your own yoga practice.

Enjoy your practice!

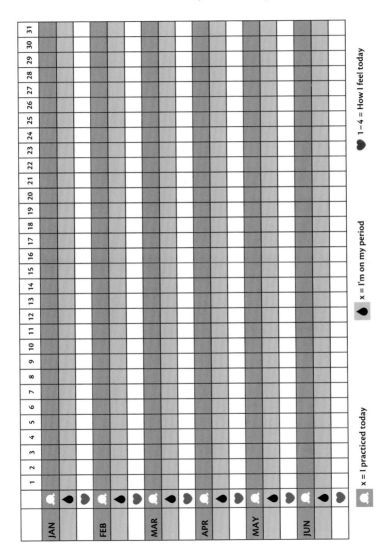

	1	2	3	4	5	6	7	8	9	10	11	12	13	14	15	16	17	18	19	20	21	22	23	24	25	26	27	28	29	30	31
JAN																															
FEB																															
MAR																															
APR																															
MAY																															
JUN																															

x = I practiced today   x = I'm on my period   1 – 4 = How I feel today

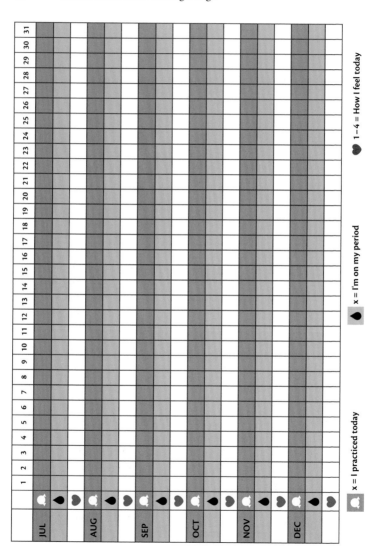

	1	2	3	4	5	6	7	8	9	10	11	12	13	14	15	16	17	18	19	20	21	22	23	24	25	26	27	28	29	30	31
JUL																															
AUG																															
SEP																															
OCT																															
NOV																															
DEC																															

x = I practiced today

x = I'm on my period

1 – 4 = How I feel today

Index

Exercises Arranged by English Name

Exercises Arranged by Sanskrit Name

Exercises Arranged by Area Helped

About the Author

Claudia Turske, born in 1953 in Zurich, has always had a strong sense of curiosity and a desire to learn. She followed this passion from a young age and decided to study anthropology, history, and political science at the University of Zurich, where she received her PhD in the 1980s. She completed additional certification as a nutritionist and psychotherapist in the 1990s.

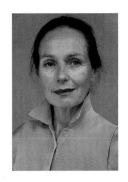

Since 1995 she has focused extensively on yoga, and in 2000 she met her first Anusara Yoga teacher in the United States. She completed her training as a yoga teacher with John Friend, the founder of Anusara Yoga.

Today she runs a yoga studio in Berlin with her husband, Vilas V. Turske; the studio trains Anusara Yoga teachers as well as hormone yoga teachers. Presently she travels frequently and teaches workshops worldwide. Her life has been shaped by her thirst for knowledge and her keen interest in people, aspects that form the basis for her investigation of various facets of yoga: breathing, meditation, asanas, and the study of philosophy. She also maintains a nutrition and psychotherapy practice in Berlin.

Lalleshvari (Turske's spiritual name) is the first certified German-speaking Anusara Yoga teacher, and she is also a hormone yoga teacher certified by Dinah Rodrigues. She has built on Rodrigues's method through years of working with many different women, adding in the proven biomechanical principles of alignment. Furthermore she is RYT 500 registered at Yoga Alliance.

The author's German-language DVD *Hormonyoga at Home* provides a specific, comprehensive set of exercise instructions. The DVD was issued by parapara and can be ordered by contacting buero .parapara@googlemail.com.